TOFU COOKBOOK

Over 30 Top Tofu Recipes For A Light Vegan Meal

BY KATYA JOHANSSON

TABLE OF CONTENTS

INTRODUCTION

Originated in China almost 2000 years ago, Tofu is made from curdled soybean milk, and has a pale white color.

Tofu is an important source of protein for vegans, vegetarians and for all those who are looking for a meatless diet.

Tofu, made from soybean curds, is naturally gluten-free and low calorie, contains no cholesterol and is an excellent source of protein, iron, and calcium.

Being, made from soybean curds, it is gluten-free and low in calories, contains no cholesterol and is an excellent source of protein, iron, calcium and a lot of more minerals.

Tofu is an excellent food for dieters because it contains high amounts of proteins and low amounts of carbs which have several health benefits. Studies show that regularly eating tofu provides an equivalent amount of energy, protein, total fat, carbohydrates, alcohol and fiber as meat. Every 100 g. of tofu contains about 17.19 g of protein.

The main health benefits of tofu will show up in significantly lower total cholesterol, triglycerides and low-density lipoprotein (bad cholesterol).

RECIPES FOR BREAKFAST

1. TOFU SCRAMBLE

INGREDIENTS:

- 1/2 red onion finely chopped
- 1/4 red bell pepper finely chopped
- 1 clove garlic minced
- 14oz extra firm tofu
- 2 teaspoons extra virgin olive oil (divided)
- 2 tablespoons nutritional yeast flakes
- 2 tablespoons McKay's vegan chicken style seasoning
- 1/8 teaspoon turmeric
- salt to taste

METHOD:

1. Place your chopped onion, bell pepper, and garlic in a skillet/frying pan with about 1 teaspoon of olive oil and sauté it on the stove on medium-high heat.
2. Remove from heat when the onions are beginning to change color.
3. Set the whole thing aside.
4. In a bowl crumble the tofu and mix in the seasonings.

5. Pour 1 teaspoon of olive oil on the bottom of a frying pan/skillet and place on your stove on medium to medium-high heat.
6. Dump the tofu on top of the olive oil, and give it a little stir.
7. Continue stirring every minute or so until your tofu begins to get firm around the edges.
8. Gently fold the onion/pepper mixture into your tofu.
9. Serve hot with salsa.

2. Tofu Scramble Ranchero

Ingredients:

- 1 tablespoon olive oil
- 1 onion, diced
- 1 green bell pepper, diced
- 2 cloves garlic, minced
- 2 jalapeños, minced (see tip)
- 1 teaspoon cumin
- 1/2 teaspoon salt, or to taste
- 1 1/2 pounds tomatoes, diced
- 1/2 cup vegetable broth
- 2 pounds extra firm tofu, drained
- 1/4 cup nutritional yeast
- 1 tablespoon prepared yellow mustard
- 1 teaspoon turmeric
- 1 teaspoon garlic powder
- 2 teaspoons onion powder
- 2 teaspoons sea salt
- freshly ground pepper
- 2 tablespoons olive oil
- 1 can black beans, drained and rinsed
- chopped fresh cilantro, vegan sour cream and warm tortillas

Method:

1. Prepare the ranchero sauce: heat olive oil in a large saucepan over medium heat.
2. Add the onion and bell pepper and cook 5-7 minutes or until tender.
3. Add the garlic, jalapeños, cumin and salt and cook 1 minute longer.
4. Add the tomatoes and cook for 2 minutes.
5. Add the vegetable broth and simmer vigorously for 15-20 minutes or until thickened.
6. Prepare the tofu: crumble the tofu to desired size in a large bowl.
7. Mash in nutritional yeast, mustard, spices, salt and pepper until well mixed.
8. Heat 2 tablespoons of olive oil in a large pan over medium heat.
9. Add the tofu mixture, and then stir in the black beans.
10. Cook, stirring occasionally, for 5 minutes or until heated through.
11. Divide tofu mixture on to plates and cover in ranchero sauce.
12. Sprinkle with chopped cilantro and serve with vegan sour cream and warm tortillas.

3. Tofu and Pinto Bean

Ingredients:

- 1 tablespoon extra-virgin olive oil
- 1 1/2 cup onion, diced
- 1/4 cup peppers (I used yellow and orange), diced
- 3 cloves garlic, finely diced
- 1 14-ounce block extra-firm tofu, pressed, drained and cubed
- 1 tablespoon sriracha (or other hot sauce)
- 1 cup mushrooms, chopped into large pieces
- 3 cups fingerling or small red potatoes, cubed
- 1 cup vegetable broth
- 3 ounces tomato paste
- 1 15-ounce can pinto beans (I used no-salt added beans), rinsed and drained
- 1 teaspoon iodized sea salt
- 1/2 teaspoon ground black pepper

Method:

1. Heat olive oil in an uncovered pressure cooker on medium-high heat.
2. Sauté onion, peppers and garlic for 3 – 5 minutes.
3. Add tofu and sriracha and sauté until the tofu has browned.
4. Add mushrooms, potatoes, vegetable broth and tomato paste, stir well, and lock the pressure cooker lid in place.

5. Bring to pressure.
6. Cook at pressure for 6 minutes.
7. Use the quick release method.
8. Remove the pressure cooker lid, away from you.
9. You will notice some amount of liquid.
10. Add the pinto beans (drained), salt and pepper to the uncovered pressure cooker.
11. Bring the hash to a boil, then reduce heat to low and simmer (the pressure cooker is still uncovered!) until the liquid cooks up
12. Serve with hot sauce, or any garnish.

4. TOFU AND VEGETABLE DISH

INGREDIENTS:

- 1 large knob Coconut Oil
- 2 cloves Garlic, chopped
- 3 medium Potatoes, diced
- 1 1/2 cups Water
- 1 head Cauliflower, cut into florets
- 1 1/2 teaspoons Ginger
- 2 teaspoons Curry
- 1/2 teaspoon Turmeric
- 1/2 teaspoon Dry Mustard
- 1/2 teaspoon Onion Powder
- 1/2 teaspoon Salt
- 1 block extra-firm Tofu, drained and diced
- 1 cup Peas

METHOD:

1. Heat the oil in a large skillet. Add the garlic and sauté over medium heat until fragrant and golden.
2. While garlic is cooking, dice potatoes. Then, add potatoes and water.
3. Cover and bring to a simmer, then cook over medium heat for 5 minutes.
4. While potatoes are cooking, chop cauliflower. Add cauliflower, ginger, curry turmeric, mustard and onion powder and continue to simmer for 5 minutes.

5. Add tofu and peas, and cook over medium heat for more 10 minutes longer, stirring occasionally.

5. TOFU PANCAKES

INGREDIENTS:

- 50g Brazil nuts
- 1 sliced banana
- berries, to serve
- maple syrup or honey, to serve
- For the batter: 349 g. pack firm silken tofu
- 2 teaspoon vanilla extract
- 2 teaspoon lemon juice
- 400ml unsweetened almond milk
- 1 tablespoon vegetable oil, plus 1-2 tablespoons extra for frying
- 250g buckwheat flour
- 4 tablespoon sugar
- 1½ teaspoon ground mixed spice
- 1 tablespoon gluten-free baking powder

METHOD:

1. Heat oven to 180C/160C fan/gas 4.
2. Scatter the nuts over a baking tray and cook for 5 mins until toasty and golden.
3. Leave to cool, then chop.
4. Turn the oven down low in order to keep the whole batch of pancakes warm.
5. Put the tofu, vanilla, lemon juice and 200ml of the milk into a deep jug or bowl. Using a stick blender, blend

together until liquid, and keep going until it turns thick and smooth, like yogurt.

6. Stir in the oil and the rest of the milk to loosen the mixture.
7. Put the dry ingredients and 1 teaspoon salt in a large bowl and whisk to combine and aerate.
8. Make a well in the center, pour in the tofu mix and bring together to make a thick batter.
9. Heat a large non-stick frying pan and swirl around 1 teaspoon oil.,
10. The pan and oil should be hot enough a sizzle on contact with the batter, but not so hot that it scorches it. Test a drop.
11. Using a ladle or large serving spoon, drop in 3 spoonful's of batter, easing it out gently in the pan.
12. Cook for 2 minutes on the first side or until bubbles pop over most of the surface.
13. Loosen with a palette knife, then flip over the pancakes and cook for 1 min more or until puffed up and firm.
14. Transfer to the oven to keep warm, but don't stack the pancakes too closely.
15. Cook the rest of the batter, using a little more oil each time.
16. Serve warm with sliced banana, berries, toasted nuts and a drizzle of maple syrup or honey.

6. TOFU OMELET

INGREDIENTS:

- 2 cloves garlic
- 1 14 oz. package silken tofu, lightly drained
- 2 tablespoons nutritional yeast
- 2 tablespoons olive oil
- 1/2 teaspoon turmeric
- 1 teaspoon sea salt, plus extra for sprinkling
- 1/2 cup chickpea flour
- 1 tablespoon arrowroot or cornstarch

METHOD:

1. Chop up the garlic up in a food processor. Add the tofu, nutritional yeast, olive oil, turmeric and salt.
2. Puree until smooth. Add the chickpea flour and cornstarch and puree again for about 10 seconds, until combined. Make sure to scrape down the sides so that everything is well incorporated.
3. Preheat a large, heavy bottomed, non-stick skillet over medium-high heat
4. Lightly grease with either cooking spray or a very thin layer of oil.
5. Use a large skillet, as you need room to spread out the omelet and to get your spatula under there to flip.
6. In 1/2 cup measurements, pour omelet batter into skillet. Use the back of a spoon or a rubber spatula to spread the batter out into about 6- inch circles.

7. Let cook for about 3 to 5 minutes before flipping. The top of the omelet should dry and become a dull matte yellow when ready to flip.
8. If you begin to flip it and it seems like it might fall apart, give it a little more time. When the omelet is ready to be flipped, the underside should be flecked with light to dark brown when it is ready to flip.
9. Flip omelet and cook for about a minute on the other side.
10. Keep warm on a plate covered with tin foil as you make the remaining omelets.
11. Stuff omelet with the fillings of your choice then fold over.
12. Once the omelet has been filled, sprinkle with a little extra sea salt.

7. Apple Cinnamon Tofu

Ingredients:

1 Block Silken Tofu with all the water

⅔ C. Date Paste (or other sweetener)

½ C. Gluten-Free All-Purpose Flour (or Wheat Flour)

2 Tablespoons Melted Coconut Oil, plus additional for greasing the pan

1½ Teaspoon Baking Powder

2 C. Chopped Apple (you can peel the apple if you like)

¼ C. Ground Flaxseeds (or Wheat Germ)

¼ C. Hemp Seeds (or use additional Ground Flaxseeds or Wheat Germ)

Cinnamon for Sprinkling

Method:

1. Pre-heat the oven to 375 degrees F.
2. Lightly grease a 10 inch pie pan or casserole dish and set aside.

3. In a blender, add the tofu with water, date paste, flour, melted coconut oil, and baking powder and blend until smooth.
4. Transfer the tofu mixture to a large bowl and stir in the chopped apple, ground flaxseeds, and hemp seeds.
5. Pour the mixture into the prepared baking dish and generously sprinkle the top with cinnamon.
6. Bake for 40-45 minutes, until the top has browned and it feels mostly firm to the touch.
7. Allow to cool and set for 5-10 minutes.
8. Serve warm.

8. SKILLET TOFU

INGREDIENTS:

- 1 block tofu, firm
- 1 tablespoon walnut oil
- 2 teaspoons oregano
- 1 clove minced garlic
- 4 halved tomatoes
- Walnuts for topping

METHOD:

1. Drain and slice tofu into large pieces.
2. Pat dry with paper towel.
3. Drizzle tofu with walnut oil and sprinkle with oregano while you warm a cast iron skillet.
4. Add more oil to pan and sear tofu on both sides.
5. Remove from pan to platter.
6. Toss in garlic and fry tomatoes for 1 minute on each side.
7. Serve with walnuts.

TOFU RECIPES FOR LUNCH

9. TASTY TOFU BOWL

INGREDIENTS:

- 350 grams firm tofu
- 80 grams low-sodium soy sauce
- 15 grams sriracha
- 40 grams maple syrup

METHOD:

1. Mix soy sauce, maple syrup and sriracha in an airtight container.
2. Cut tofu into desired shape and don't drain it.
3. Mix tofu with the marinade.
4. Chill on the fridge for at least 5-6 hours (overnight is best!)
5. Heat some oil in a pan and stir fry until tofu looks crispy and golden.
6. Serve with sautéed zucchini, steamed broccoli, baked sweet potato fries, leafy greens salad with tahini with lemon juice.

10. Noodles with Stir-Fried Tofu and Vegetables

Ingredients:

8 oz. dried rice vermicelli

4 Tablespoon vegetable oil

8 oz. firm tofu, drained and cut into rectangular strips about 1-inch wide

2 shallots, thinly sliced

6 dried black mushrooms, soaked in hot water for 30 min., drained, stemmed, and thinly sliced

2 cups broccoli florets cut through their stems into thin slices, stewed in boiling water and drained

1-1/2 cups shredded green or Napa cabbage

1-1/2 cups thinly sliced bok choy

2 Tablespoons soy sauce; more or less to taste

1/2 red bell pepper, thinly sliced

2 cups washed and shredded romaine, red, or green leaf lettuce

2 cups fresh, crisp bean sprouts

1-1/2 cups peeled, seeded, and julienned cucumber

1/3 to 1/2 cup roughly chopped or small whole mint leaves

1/3 to 1/2 cup roughly chopped or small basil or Thai basil leaves

2 Tablespoons chopped roasted peanuts

12 sprigs fresh cilantro

1 recipe Vietnamese Dipping Sauce (Nuoc Cham)

METHOD:

1. Cook the noodles:
2. Cook the tofu and vegetables:
3. Heat 2 Tbs. of the oil in a nonstick pan or skillet over medium heat.
4. Add the tofu pieces and stir-fry until nicely browned.
5. Remove and drain on paper towels. When cool, cut them into bite-size strips.
6. Set aside.
7. Heat the remaining oil in a large skillet or sauté pan over high heat. Wait until the oil gets very hot, almost smoking (the vegetables should sizzle during the entire cooking time), and add the shallots, constantly stirring until they become fragrant, about 20 seconds.
8. Add the mushrooms and stir-fry for another 20 seconds.
9. Add the broccoli, cabbage, and bok choy, stir for 30 seconds, and add the red bell pepper. (, sprinkle in 1 to 2 Tbs. water if the pan gets dry.
10. Quickly, create an open space in the middle of the pan by pushing the vegetables against the edges.
11. Add the soy sauce to the open area. It should sizzle and caramelize slightly, creating a distinctive aroma.

12. Stir the vegetables with the soy sauce a few times and remove from the heat.
13. Toss the vegetables with the tofu.
14. Assemble the salads: divide the lettuce, bean sprouts, cucumber, mint, and basil among four large soup or pasta bowls. Fluff the noodles with your fingers and divide them among the prepared salad bowls.
15. Put the tofu and vegetables over the noodles and garnish each bowl with the peanuts and cilantro.
16. Pass the nuoc cham at the table; each diner should drizzle about 3 Tbs. over the salad and then toss the salad in the bowl a few times with two forks or chopsticks before eating.

11. GRILLED TOFU SKEWERS

INGREDIENTS:

- 1 container extra firm tofu, drained and sliced into large chunks
- 1 zucchini, cut into large chunks
- 1 red bell pepper, cut into large chunks
- 10 large mushrooms
- 2 tablespoons sriracha chili garlic sauce
- 1/4 cup soy sauce
- 2 tablespoons sesame oil
- 1/4 cup diced onion
- 1 jalapeno pepper, diced
- Ground black pepper to taste

METHOD:

1. Place tofu, zucchini, red bell pepper, and mushrooms in a bowl.
2. Mix sriracha sauce, soy sauce, sesame oil, onion, jalapeno, and pepper in a small bowl, and pour over tofu and vegetables.
3. Toss lightly to coat.
4. Cover, and allow marinating at least 1 hour in the refrigerator.
5. Preheat an outdoor or any grill for medium-high heat, and lightly oil the grate.
6. Thread tofu and vegetables on to skewers.
7. Grill each skewer 10 minutes, or to desired doneness.
8. Use any remaining marinade as a dipping sauce.

12. QUINOA TOFU VEGGIES

INGREDIENTS:

- 1 c quinoa
- 1/2 package extra firm tofu
- 1 - 2 Tablespoon soy sauce
- 2 Tablespoon cooking oil
- 1 Tablespoon peeled minced fresh ginger
- 1 garlic clove, minced
- 2 medium carrots
- 2 stalks celery
- 1/4 cup cashew pieces
- 1 bay leaf
- 1 teaspoon grounded coriander
- 1 teaspoon grounded fennel
- 1 medium zucchini (6 - 8 inches)
- 1/4 teaspoon dried rosemary leaf, or 1 tsp chopped fresh rosemary
- 1 teaspoon dried basil leaf
- 1 1/2 cup water
- 1/4 teaspoon salt
- 1/4 cup chopped black olives
- 1/4 c. minced parsley or cilantro

METHOD:

1. Rinse quinoa, drain and set aside.
2. Cut tofu in bite sized cubes, place in a small bowl, sprinkle with soy sauce and shake or stir to coat. Set aside.

3. Heat 1 Tbsp. olive oil on low in a large sauté pan or shallow 4 qt. sauce pan.
4. Mince ginger and garlic.
5. Chop celery in small piece.s
6. Peel and chop carrots in 1/2" dice.
7. Wash, trim, and chop zucchini in 1 " dice. Set aside.
8. Coarsely chop olives and set aside.
9. Turn the heat up to medium, and stir fry ginger, garlic, celery, carrots, and cashews for 5 minutes.
10. Add the drained quinoa and stir until dry -about 5 minutes.
11. Add dry spices, stir 1 minute.
12. Stir in zucchini, herbs, water, salt
13. Bring to a boil, cover and cook 12 minutes on low heat.
14. Fry the tofu cubes on medium in 1 Tbsp. oil stirring and turning, until browned.
15. Stir fried tofu, chopped olives and parsley or cilantro into the quinoa and veggies.
16. Heat on low for another minute and serve.

13. CHIPOTLE GREEN ONION TOFU

INGREDIENTS:

- 1 1/2 chipotle pepper with Adobo Sauce
- 2 garlic clove, minced
- 1 teaspoon lemon juice (or to taste)
- 1/2 cup vegan mayo
- 1/4 cup Silken Soft Tofu
- 1 tablespoon chives (or green onions), finely chopped
- fresh grounded black pepper

METHOD:

1. Add all the ingredients, except for the chives, into a blender.
2. For the chipotle pepper, scoop one out of the can with the Adobo sauce.
3. Blend until completely pureed into a thick and creamy aioli.
4. Pour the aioli into a bowl. Add the finely chopped chives.
5. Add some freshly ground black pepper to taste. If needed adjust the seasoning with some salt or additional lemon juice.
6. Chill in the fridge and use as a spread for sandwiches or wraps, or as a dipping sauce!

14. SMOKED TOFU PAN-FRIED DUMPLINGS

INGREDIENTS:

- 1 package round wonton wrappers
- 200g package of firm smoked tofu
- 2 Tablespoon vegetable oil
- 1 large head of cabbage, shredded finely
- 1 large onion, diced
- 2 cups of grated carrot
- 4 cloves garlic, crushed
- 4 Tablespoon fresh grated ginger
- For the dipping sauce:
- ¼ cup soy sauce
- 1 scallion, finely chopped
- 2 Tablespoon fresh chopped cilantro
- ½ cup soy sauce
- ½ cup water
- ¼ cup rice vinegar
- 1 Tablespoon sesame oil
- 2 Tablespoon brown sugar

METHOD:

1. Finely dice onion, and shred cabbage.
2. Heat oil in a large skillet over medium heat.
3. Add onions, and cook, stirring occasionally, until golden brown.

4. Add the cabbage, carrot, garlic, and ginger. Cook over medium heat, stirring frequently, until cabbage has cooked down and the filling is soft.
5. Add cubed tofu, and ¼ cup of soy sauce, and cook, for another 2 min.
6. Turn off heat and set filling aside to cool slightly.
7. Line a large baking sheet with parchment paper.
8. Set up an assembly station with a stack of wonton wrappers, a small bowl of water, and your filling. Place a wonton wrapper in one hand, and fill with about 1 Tbsp. of filling
9. Dip a finger in the bowl of water, and run your wet finger around the perimeter of the wonton wrapper. Fold in half, and pinch around the edges to seal shut. Place on the lined baking sheet. Repeat.
10. To cook the gyoza (Japanese Pan-Fried Dumplings) from fresh, heat some vegetable oil in a large skillet over medium heat.
11. Place gyoza in a single layer in the skillet, leaving sufficient room to flip.
12. Cook until golden on one side, flip, and cook until golden on the other.
13. Serve immediately, or at room temperature.
14. To make dipping sauce, whisk ingredients together in a bowl.
15. Serve.

15. INDIAN TOFU FRIED TURNOVER (SAMOSAS)

INGREDIENTS:

- 200g (or approx. half a packet) of Tofu made into a scramble, mashed with a fork
- Readymade Filo pastry sheets
- 200g of crushed broad beans/lima beans
- 1 small onion, finely chopped
- 2 tablespoons of fresh mint leaves, finely chopped
- 1 green chili, finely chopped
- 1 inch piece of ginger, finely chopped
- 1 teaspoon of garam masala
- 1 teaspoon of cumin seeds
- 1/2 teaspoons of salt
- 1 teaspoon of lemon juice
- 1 tablespoons of oil
- 30g of melted coconut oil

Method:

1. Add the 1 tablespoon of oil into a non-stick pan and then when hot add the cumin seeds, so they fizzle in the oil for about 30 seconds.
2. Add the chopped onions, ginger and chilies.
3. Mix well and sauté for about 2 minutes in the pan on a low heat.

4. Add the crushed broad beans and mix well and sauté together again for 2 mins.
5. Then add the tofu, garam masala, salt and chopped mint.
6. Mix well and sauté for about 5 mins or until most of the moisture has evaporated and the mixture is quite dry.
7. Cool the mixture completely or until you can handle it with your hands.
8. Sprinkle the lemon juice over the cooled mixture and mix well.
9. Take one pastry sheet and place on a board and brush the melted coconut oil around the edges.
10. Fold in half (lengthways) and brush the sides again. Add 3 teaspoons of the tofu filling on the top left corner of your pastry. Then fold the pastry with the filling, brushing with melted coconut oil as you go. Ensure you fold the pastry as tightly with the filling as you can, to ensure the filling will be secure when baking.
11. Do these until you finish all the filling and then brush each samosa with the oil on the outsides and place on a greaseproof baking tray.
12. Place in an oven at 200 C for 15 mins, and turn the tray half way through so the Samosa's are cooked even.

16. Tofu and Mushroom Miso Soup

INGREDIENTS:

- 6 ounces tofu, cubed
- 4 ounces fresh mushrooms, sliced
- a handful of leafy vegetable, chopped
- 1 tablespoon vegan egg
- 2 tablespoons chopped green onion
- cup s water
- tablespoons Miso & Easy

METHOD:

1. In a sauce pot, bring the broth to a boil. Add in the tofu, mushrooms and the vegetables. While stirring the broth, slowly pour in the vegan egg.
2. Cook for 2 minutes. Remove the pot from the heat.
3. If using Miso & Easy: Stir in the Miso & Easy. Top with green onions and serve immediately.
4. If using Miso Paste: Ladle about ½ cup of the hot broth into a bowl with the miso paste. Use a fork or whisk to stir, liquefy and soften the miso paste. Pour all of the miso paste into the pot and stir gently.
5. Top with green onions and serve immediately.

Tofu Recipes for Dinner

19. Ginger Garlic Tofu Recipe

INGREDIENTS:

- 1 16-ounce package of hard tofu
- 1/4 cup hot water
- 2 tablespoons palm sugar or brown sugar
- 1/2 cup dashi or cold water
- 1/2 cup soy sauce or gluten-free tamari
- 1/4 cup rice vinegar
- 1 tablespoon sesame oil
- 1 teaspoon crushed red pepper
- 2 teaspoons minced fresh ginger
- 2 teaspoons minced/grated daikon radish(optional)
- 4 cloves garlic, minced

METHOD:

1. Remove the tofu from its package.
2. Slice the tofu into smaller blocks about one half inch by 2 inches
3. Drain the blocks on clean kitchen towels or paper towels.
4. Combine the sugar and hot water and mix until the sugar is fully dissolved.

5. Combine the sugar-water with the remaining ingredients in a small bowl or container, just big enough to fit the tofu.
6. Place the tofu in the container, followed by the marinade.
7. Soak for at least four hours, (ideally overnight).
8. Remove the tofu from the marinade, then sauté, fry, grill, or steam as desired.
9. The sautéed tofu can be put on banh mi sandwiches, in noodle bowls, or fried in tempura.

20. CARAMELIZED TOFU AND BROCCOLI

INGREDIENTS:

15 oz. extra-firm tofu, or use boneless chicken or beef

2 tablespoon coconut or peanut oil

1 teaspoon minced garlic, (1 – 2 cloves)

1/2 cup pecans, coarsely chopped

2 tablespoon brown sugar

3 tablespoon reduced-sodium soy sauce

1/4 teaspoon crushed red pepper flakes

1 head broccoli, cut into florets

1/2 red bell pepper, cut into thin 1-inch long strips

1/2 red onion, thinly sliced

METHOD:

1. Drain the tofu and wrap it in a clean dishcloth to draw out the extra water.
2. Cut the tofu into 3 crosswise slices, and cut those slices into 3 or 4 long strips.

3. In a large skillet, heat the oil over medium-high heat. Add the tofu strips and cook them without stirring for about 3 minutes until they have browned on the bottom.
4. Flip the tofu and add the garlic and pecans, stirring them for a minute until the garlic becomes fragrant.
5. Add the sugar, 1 1/2 Tbsp. soy sauce, and the red pepper flakes and stir until the sugar blends with the rest of the ingredients.
6. Remove the tofu and nuts to a plate, allowing some of the sauce to remain in the pan.
7. Add the broccoli, red pepper strips, onions, and the remaining soy sauce and cook for 3 – 4 minutes until they are tender.
8. Slice the oranges; add the tofu and other ingredients back into the skillet to heat them through.
9. Serve immediately.

21. SQUASH AND TOFU

INGREDIENTS:

- (14-ounce) package extra-firm tofu, drained
- 2 pounds dumpling, or acorn squash, halved and seeded
- 1 ½ tablespoons soy sauce, or more to taste
- ½ teaspoon sriracha or other hot sauce
- Sea salt, and black pepper
- ¼ cup peanut oil
- 1 tablespoon honey
- 1 tablespoon toasted sesame seeds
- 2 tablespoons chopped celery leaves or cilantro

METHOD:

1. Drain tofu and slice into 1/2-inch-thick slabs.
2. Cut each slab in half.
3. Arrange tofu on a large baking sheet or several plates lined with several layers of paper towels.
4. Place another layer of paper towels on top and weigh down tofu with another baking sheet or more plates topped with a heavy cookbook or cans. Let stand for 20 minutes.
5. Pat tofu dry.
6. While tofu drains, heat oven to 425 degrees.
7. Cut squash into 1/2-inch-thick half-moons. Cut each slice in half again.

8. In a small bowl, whisk together soy sauce, sriracha and a pinch of salt. Whisk in peanut oil.
9. Spoon 3 tablespoons of the mixture into a separate bowl and reserve.
10. Whisk honey into the original mixture.
11. Spread squash out on a large baking sheet and pour honey-soy mixture over it.
12. Sprinkle squash lightly with salt and pepper and toss well.
13. Roast until bottoms are golden brown, about 20 minutes.
14. Flip and roast until uniformly golden and soft, about 10 minutes more.
15. Transfer squash to a large bowl.
16. Adjust the heat to broil and position a rack just below the heating element.
17. Toss tofu with reserved soy mixture and arrange in a single layer on a baking sheet.
18. Cook until crispy and golden, about 2 minutes per side.
19. Toss hot tofu with squash, sesame seeds and celery leaves, adding more soy sauce if you like.

22. TOFU WITH RICE

INGREDIENTS:

- 1 package extra-firm tofu, drained and cubed
- 1 teaspoon seasoned salt
- 1 tablespoon canola oil
- 1 small onion, chopped
- 3 garlic cloves, minced
- 1/2 cup light coconut milk
- 1/4 cup minced fresh cilantro
- 1 teaspoon curry powder
- 1/4 teaspoon salt
- 1/4 teaspoon pepper
- 2 cups cooked brown rice

METHOD:

1. Sprinkle tofu with seasoned salt.
2. In a large nonstick skillet coated with cooking spray, sauté tofu in oil until lightly browned. Remove and keep warm.
3. In the same skillet, sauté onion and garlic for 1-2 minutes or until crisp-tender.
4. Stir in the coconut milk, cilantro, curry, salt and pepper.
5. Bring to a boil.
6. Reduce heat; simmer, uncovered, for 4-5 minutes or until sauce is slightly thickened.

7. Stir in tofu; heat through.
8. Serve with rice.

23. TOFU STIR FRY

INGREDIENTS:

- 2 tablespoon, vegetable Oil
- Tofu 450 g, in cubes
- 4 each Shallot
- 2 cloves garlic, crushed
- 1 tablespoon, fresh Ginger
- 200 g, mini cobs Corn
- 200 g, snow Peas
- 200 g. snow Peas
- 200 g, shitake Mushrooms
- 225 ml Vegetable stock
- 1 tablespoon, brown Sugar
- 1 tablespoon, Soy sauce
- 2 tablespoon Cornstarch

METHOD:

1. In a nonstick skillet, heat 1 teaspoon vegetable oil over medium-high heat until hot.
2. Add tofu, and cook, about 4 minutes, gently tossing until heated through and lightly golden.
3. Transfer to plate; set aside.
4. Meanwhile, heat remaining 1 teaspoon vegetable oil in a large wok.
5. Add the shallots, garlic, ginger, corn, snow peas, beansprouts and mushrooms.

6. Cook for 5 minutes, stirring frequently.
7. Add the tofu to wok.
8. Pour in the stock, sugar, soy sauce and cornstarch.
9. Heat to boiling and cook for 2 minutes to heat and thicken.

24. TOFU AND POTATO LATKES

INGREDIENTS:

- 14 ounces (400 g) peeled and grated potato
- 8 ounces (240 g) grated super-firm tofu
- 3 tablespoons vegan egg
- 1 1/2 tablespoons cornstarch
- 3/4 teaspoon sea salt
- 1 teaspoon black pepper
- 1/2 cup finely chopped green onion
- 6 tablespoons coconut oil
- 6 tablespoons canola oil

METHOD:

1. Put the potato in a bowl, add water to cover, swish, and drain.
2. Wring out in clean muslin or a dishtowel.
3. Transfer to a clean dishtowel.
4. Repeat with the tofu and add to the potato.
5. Let sit at room temperature or in a warm oven for 1 1/2 to 2 hours to dry out, until it's no longer wet.
6. In a large bowl, beat together the vegan eggs, cornstarch, salt, and pepper.
7. Add the potato, tofu and green onion. Mix well. Set near the stove with a baking sheet with a rack or paper towel placed inside.

8. Heat half of the coconut butter and oil in a large skillet over medium-high heat. The bottom of the skillet should be filmed.
9. Scoop up about 2 lightly packed tablespoons of the latke mixture and place in the skillet.
10. Pat and gently flatten into patties about 3/8 inch thick and 2 1/2 inches wide.
11. Repeat to form more in the skillet. Don't over crowd them. Fry for 2 to 3 minutes per side, until richly brown and crisp.
12. Cool on the rack or paper towel.
13. Add a little more coconut butter and oil to the skillet and return the skillet to temperature (lower the heat, if needed) and fry more.
14. Repeat until all the latke mixture is used.
15. Keep the fried ones warm in the oven, if needed.
16. Serve warm with toppings.

25. TOFU CHILAQUILAS

INGREDIENTS:

- 5 small yellow corn tortillas
- 1/2 large white onion, diced
- 2 cloves garlic, minced
- 1 15 ounce can crushed tomatoes or tomato sauce
- 1 chipotle in adobo (canned) + 1 tablespoon of preferred sauce
- 1/2 cup veggie stock
- 8 ounces extra firm tofu, drained and pressed in a clean towel for 15 minutes
- •1/2 tsp cumin
- •1/2 teaspoon garlic powder
- •1/4 teaspoon chili powder
- •1/4 teaspoon sea salt
- •Diced onion and/or Fresh Cilantro
- •Salsa or hot sauce
- •Lime juice

METHOD:

1. Start by quickly pressing/draining your tofu in a clean kitchen towel with a heavy pot on top and preheating oven to 350 degrees F.
2. Stack and cut tortillas into triangles and arrange in a single layer on a large baking sheet.

3. Bake for 10-12 minutes, flipping once halfway through, until crisp and just slightly golden brown. Set aside.
4. If using regular chips, skip this step.
5. While chips are baking, heat a large skillet over medium heat and prepare onion and garlic.
6. Once hot, add 1 Tbsp. olive or canola oil and onion. Cook, stirring frequently, until soft and slightly browned. Then add garlic and cook for 1-2 minutes more.
7. Add tomato sauce, diced chipotle and adobo sauce, and veggie stock. Heat until bubbly, and then reduce heat to low and simmer for 5 minutes.
8. Transfer sauce to a blender and blend well.
9. Use a fork to crumble the tofu and place skillet back over medium heat
10. Add a bit of oil to the pan and then add tofu.
11. Let lightly brown for 3-4 minutes, stirring once or twice.
12. Then add seasonings (chili powder, salt, garlic powder and cumin) and stir.
13. Cook for another 2 minutes, then remove from pan and set aside.
14. Add chips to the pan and pour over sauce, stirring quickly to coat.
15. Then top with tofu scramble, fresh onion and cilantro and serve immediately.
16. Additional toppings might include hot sauce, lime juice, salsa .

26. Crispy Barbequed Tofu

Ingredients:

- 1 (16 ounce) package extra firm tofu
- 3 tablespoons olive oil
- 1 tablespoon egg substitute
- 1 tablespoon barbeque sauce
- 1 cup all-purpose flour
- 1 teaspoon salt
- 1/2 teaspoon pepper
- 1 cup barbeque sauce

Method:

1. Drain tofu, and slice into strips. Place in a plastic bag or container, and freeze overnight. This will give the tofu a meatier texture.
2. Thaw tofu strips, and blot with paper towels to dry.
3. Heat olive oil in a large skillet over medium heat.
4. In a small bowl, whisk together the egg substitute and 1 tablespoon of barbeque sauce.
5. Combine the flour, salt, and pepper in a separate bowl.
6. Dip the tofu slices into the vegan egg mixture, then into the flour mixture, shaking off excess flour.
7. Fry in the hot oil for about 1 minute on each side, until golden brown.
8. Just fry that much at once so they are not crowded. Remove from the oil to paper towels to drain and cool.
9. Preheat the oven's broiler.

10. Brush tofu slices with additional barbeque sauce, and allow marinating while the broiler heats up.
11. Arrange them on a broiler pan, or wire rack set over a cookie sheet for best results.
12. Position the oven rack about 6 inches from the heat source.
13. Broil for 5 minutes on each side, or until browned and crisp, watching closely so as not to burn them.
14. Serve warm with the remaining barbeque sauce for dipping.

TOFU RECIPES FOR DESSERT

27. CHOCOLATE PUDDING

INGREDIENTS:

- 19 ounces silken tofu
- 2 tablespoon raw cacao powder)
- 3-4 tablespoon agave syrup
- 1-2 tablespoon light coconut milk
- 1/4 tsp pink salt
- Fresh fruit: I added fresh organic raspberries and one sliced banana.

METHOD:

1. Add all the ingredients to your blender.
2. Blend and serve.
3. You can also make this ahead of time and chill in fridge until ready to serve.

28. SWEET TOFU WITH VANILLA

INGREDIENTS:

200 g of cookies

•125 g of coconut butter, melted

•900 grams of silken tofu type

•125 ml of maple syrup

•1 teaspoon of vanilla essence

•2 teaspoons of lemon juice

METHOD:

1. Preheat the oven to 180 º C.
2. Make the crust, place cookies and coconut butter in a blender and shred until it crumble.
3. Place in a greased tray and refrigerate.
4. To make the filling, crumble tofu in a blender cup.
5. Add the remaining ingredients and beat until a smooth texture.
6. Pour the mixture into the biscuit base and bake for 35-40 minutes.

29. Vanilla Ice Cream

Ingredients:

- 1 cup silken tofu mixed with 1 ¼ cup non-dairy milk
- About 1 cup raw, unsalted cashews with 2 ½ cups water, simmered, covered for 15 minutes or soaked for 12 hours
- 2 Tablespoons + 2 teaspoons vegetable oil
- ½ cup + 2 Tablespoons sugar
- ⅓ cup corn syrup or agave syrup
- 2 teaspoons unrefined coconut oil, melted
- 1 teaspoon cocoa butter, melted ½ teaspoon apple cider vinegar
- ¼ teaspoon salt
- 2 vanilla beans, or 1 Tablespoon vanilla extract
- ½ teaspoon xanthan gum

Method:

1. If you're using tofu as a base: place it in a blender with the non-dairy milk. It's important to not use boxed tofu like Mori-Nu. These types of tofu inhibit the ice cream's ability to harden properly.
2. Cashew Base: place the soaked or simmered cashews along with their water in a blender.
3. Blend the ice cream ingredients.

4. Place the vegetable oil, sugar, corn syrup, coconut oil, cocoa butter, apple cider vinegar and salt into the blender. If using vanilla beans, cut the vanilla beans in half lengthwise and scrape out the paste. Add the vanilla paste to the blender and discard the outer bean halves. If you're not using vanilla beans, add the vanilla extract.
5. Place the lid on the blender and place a towel over the top to protect against spillover.
6. Blend on low for 1 minute.
7. While the blender is running, carefully remove the small top cap of the blender and pour the xanthan gum into the blender vortex and blend an additional 1 minute.
8. Transfer the mixture to a bowl and place it in the refrigerator until completely cold, about 4 hours.
9. Process the vegan ice cream in an ice cream maker then transfer to the freezer to harden.
10. Process the mixture in an ice cream maker for 30 minutes. If you're planning on adding any chopped ingredients, add them to the ice cream maker during the last 3 minutes.
11. While the mixture is processing, chill your ice cream container in the freezer. This will ensure that the ice cream is as cold as possible as it goes into the freezer.
12. Transfer the ice cream to the container, packing it down to make sure there are as few air pockets as possible.
13. Chill for at least 12 hours.

30. BERRY TOFU PUDDING

INGREDIENTS:

- 12 oz. of fresh raspberries and blueberries in equal quantities
- 5 tablespoons filtered water
- 5 tablespoons pure maple syrup
- 1 teaspoon lemon juice plus more to taste
- 1 packet (12 oz./300 grams) package of organic firm silken tofu
- Pinch Celtic sea salt, plus more to taste

METHOD:

1. Put berries in a saucepan with the water and sweetener, bring to the boil, and then lower the heat, and simmer until tender and a syrup forms.
2. Cool.
3. Put everything in your blender with the berries, and blast on high until smooth and creamy.
4. Add in more lemon juice and sweetener to taste if desired.
5. Chill in the fridge, and serve topped with more fresh berries and vegan cream.

31. TOFU CHEESECAKE

INGREDIENTS:

FOR THE BATTER:
- 1 cup cashews, soaked
- 6-ounce (175g) silken tofu
- 1 tablespoon peanut butter
- 1 small banana
- A handful of shredded coconut
- Pinch of sea salt
- 1-ounce (30ml) water
- 2 tablespoons raw cacao powder blend into half of the batter

FOR THE SWIRE:
- 1 tablespoon peanut butter
- 1 teaspoon agave syrup

MIX AT THE END
- 3 tablespoons raisins, soaked in rum
- 4 figs, chopped

METHOD:

1. Soak raisins in rum.
2. Soak cashews in water for 2- 2.5 hours.
3. Rinse and drain.

4. Throw the ingredients in the batter ingredients (except cacao powder) into blender.
5. Blend until smooth batter forms.
6. Now, put half of the mixture into a bowl and add cacao powder to the half in the blender.
7. Mix half of raisins and chopped figs into brown batter and the other half into white batter.
8. Prepare the swirl by mixing together peanut butter (room temperature) and agave syrup.
9. Now, start compiling the bowls: Put brown and white batter into bowls by turns. Add small balls of peanut butter mix here and there.
10. When you come to the last layer, add about 5 peanut butter balls on top.
11. Take sushi stick and make some nice swirls on top of the dessert.
12. Place the desserts in fridge for a few hours.
13. Cover the bowls with foil if you need to keep them longer.

31. TOFU PUMPKIN PIE

INGREDIENTS:

- 1 can pureed pumpkin
- 3/4 cup sugar or 1/2 cup maple syrup
- 1 package silken soft tofu
- 2 to 3 tablespoons cornstarch
- 1 teaspoon ground allspice
- 1 teaspoon ground cinnamon
- 1/2 teaspoon ground ginger
- 1/2 teaspoon ground nutmeg
- 1/2 teaspoon salt
- 1/4 teaspoon ground cloves
- 1 unbaked vegan pie shell

METHOD:

1. Preheat oven to 425 degrees Fahrenheit.
2. Blend the pumpkin and sugar.
3. Thoroughly mix in tofu, cornstarch, and spices
4. Pour mixture into pie shell and bake for 15 minutes.
5. Lower heat to 350 degrees Fahrenheit and bake for another 60 minutes.
6. Chill and serve.

32. TOFU AND BLUEBERRIES

INGREDIENTS:

TOFU CREAM:
- 1 pack silken tofu
- 1/3 cup rice syrup
- 1 tablespoon olive, sunflower or safflower oil
- 1 tablespoon soymilk
- 1 ½ teaspoon vanilla extract
- 1 teaspoon lemon juice

BLUEBERRY SAUCE:
- 4 cups fresh blueberries (use frozen if not in season)
- 1/3 cup rice syrup
- 1 tablespoon lemon juice
- 2 tablespoon kuzu (gluten free starch)

METHOD:

1. Tofu Cream: whip all ingredients together in a blender until very smooth.
2. Refrigerate at least two hours before serving.
3. Blueberry Sauce: Set aside one cup of the blueberries for topping the dessert.
4. Place the remaining 3 cups of blueberries in a pot with the rice syrup and lemon juice.
5. Dissolve the kuzu in two tablespoons of water and add to the pot.
6. Bring to a boil and simmer on low heat for 4 minutes.

7. Stir in the kuzu and simmer until the mixture starts to thicken.
8. Transfer to a blender and blend to a cream.
9. Pour into a bowl and allow cooling.
10. Chill in the refrigerator for at least two hours.
11. Use glasses and layer some blueberry sauce in the bottom and tofu cream on top.
12. Continue this process of layering until the glass is full, and then top with blueberries and toasted flaked almonds, or nuts of your choice.
13. Allow two hours for chilling both the Tofu Cream and the Blueberry Sauce.

33. FRENCH TOFU STICKS

INGREDIENTS:

- 1 block tofu, extra firm
- 2 tablespoon stevia (or other sweetener)
- 1/2 tablespoon cinnamon
- For the chocolate syrup: 1.5 tablespoon coconut oil, melted
- 1 tablespoon cacao powder
- A few drops liquid stevia to taste

METHOD:

1. Drain tofu: wrap block of tofu in paper towel.
2. Place cutting board on top of the block of tofu.
3. Apply even pressure to the top of the block by placing a weight on top of the cutting board.
4. Let tofu drain for about 15-20 minutes.
5. While tofu is draining, combine cinnamon and stevia in mixing bowl to make the cinnamon-sugar topping.
6. When tofu is done draining, cut into uniform sticks.
7. Spray frypan with cooking spray and heat on low heat.
8. Flip tofu every 3-4 minutes for about 30 minutes, or until firm to the touch.
9. Halfway through, sprinkle cinnamon-sugar on the top and bottom sides of the tofu.
10. When the tofu is finished, prepare chocolate syrup.
11. Heat coconut oil in microwave for 30 seconds to 1 minute until it liquefies.

12. Add cacao powder and stevia to the coconut oil and mix thoroughly.
13. Drizzle chocolate syrup on top of the tofu sticks and serve.

Printed in Poland
by Amazon Fulfillment
Poland Sp. z o.o., Wrocław